Bind Us Together

Supplemental Activities for the Christian Initiation of Adults into the Catholic Church

by

Gerard P. Weber and
Robert L. Miller

Bind us together, Lord,
bind us together with cords that cannot be broken.

From the hymn, *Bind Us Together*, by B. Gillman

ACTA Publications
Chicago, Illinois

Bind Us Together:
Supplemental Activities for the Christian Initiation of Adults into the Catholic Church

by Rev. Gerard P. Weber and Rev. Robert L. Miller

Fr. Weber, a priest of the Archdiocese of Chicago, is an author, editor and religious educator. Fr. Miller, of the diocese of San Bernardino, is an author, theologian, counselor and retreat director. Both priests have extensive experience in parish ministry.

Edited by Nancy Benvenga and Gregory F. Augustine Pierce

Artwork by Isz

Design and Typography by Garrison Publications

Library of Congress Number: 92-075790

ISBN: 0-87946-082-2

Printed in the United States of America

CONTENTS

Introduction

The liturgical rites of the Order of Christian Initiation of Adults are steps by which the church community accepts candidates into full membership. In many parishes, unfortunately, it is difficult for newly baptized Catholics to find fellowship and friendship in the church after the conclusion of the initiation process, if they do not already have a network of Catholic friends.

The activities in Section I of *Bind Us Together* are intended to help the members of a particular initiation group build support and acceptance of one another as the candidates journey toward Baptism. These activities are designed to "bind" all the participants (candidates, leaders, sponsors) together in such a way that the candidates will have a natural support group of Catholic friends after they are baptized. Each of these simple activities is designed to be held at the time of one of the major steps in the process of Christian initiation.

The activities in Section II of this book are introductory exercises to be used in conjunction with the study of the major doctrinal questions in the catechesis process. They are intended to help participants reflect on their faith experiences, as well as to give the leaders and sponsors an indication of how the candidates think and feel about various subjects.

In both sections, some of the activities require Activity Sheets, which are provided in Section III on separate pages that may be duplicated.

Bind Us Together is not intended to be a systematic program of activities for the Christian Initiation of Adults. Groups are encouraged to select as many or as few of the activities that they feel suit their needs. (For example, some of the activities work better with well-educated people, while others are more successful with less formally educated people. Some activities take but a few moments, others longer. Most require materials prepared ahead of time; some require no supplies at all.)

Thus, it is not intended that all the activities in *Bind Us Together* be used by any one group. The facilitators or leaders will need to go through the book ahead of time and select those that seem most appropriate for the participants. A good number of the activities can also be used with slight modifications on occasions or with topics other than those indicated.

Each of the activities in *Bind Us Together* calls upon a different aspect of the participants' faith lives. Some call for them to share their *experiences* in a certain area. Others probe their *ideas* about a topic, and still others ask them to express their *feelings* about a subject. Because it is impossible to predict which direction the discussions will take, leaders will have to synthesize the discussions with the points being made in the initiation process. If this is not done, the activities will not serve their purpose.

Leaders should allow sufficient time for everyone to complete each activity. If a group is small, everyone can share his or her comments with the entire group. If the group (including leaders and sponsors) contains more than seven people, it is best to split into two or more groups of four or five people each whenever "small group" discussion or activity is called for. If there is time, the small groups may make *brief* reports to the entire group on the tenor of their sharing or what they learned from the activity.

A few activities may require more time than the leaders feel can be allotted to it during a session. In this case, it is suggested that group members do the exercise ahead of time and come to the session prepared to share their results.

Note: Throughout the book the word "participants" rather than "candidates" is used, because in many groups people other than the candidates will be in regular attendance. This is a spiritual growth process for them as well as for the people seeking to join the church.

Directions

Three simple rules of procedure will help to ensure that the sharing and the discussions stimulated by the activities in *Bind Us Together* are profitable for all. Present these instructions to the entire group at the beginning of the first activity and gently but firmly remind the participants of them whenever necessary during other activities.

1. *Allow equal time for all persons.* When an activity requires that the participants divide into small groups, everyone in the small group should have an opportunity to talk. If fifteen minutes are allotted for discussion and five people are in each group, for example, each person should be allowed approximately three minutes to share his or her thoughts or feelings.

2. *Respect what each person says.* People are expressing their ideas, feelings and experiences. These should be respected and accepted without criticism. No one in the group should argue with or try to correct ideas with which they do not agree; nor should they preach, lecture or offer advice to others in the group. Do not chide people if they have no response or, in those cases where factual answers are called for, if they give an incorrect answer. There will be times when a person in a group may feel uncomfortable or embarrassed about responding to a particular question. At all times people are free to say, "I pass."

3. *Speak for yourself.* Do not talk about other people's actions or ideas. Speak in the first person about your own ideas, your feelings, your experiences: "*I* think, *I* feel, *my* experience has been . . ."

Finally, several of the activities are "right-brain" (artistic) rather than "left-brain" (reasoning) activities. Some people feel uneasy doing activities that call more on intuition than reasoning. Assure them that using images and feelings reveals aspects and depths of an experience that logical analysis and reasoning can easily miss.

SECTION I

Activities to Build Community

The people who come to join the church are from many different backgrounds. Some are young, some not so young. Some are highly educated, others lack much formal education. Some are professional people, others are blue-collar workers. Some are happily married, some are single, some have known the pain of divorce. Some have been committed adherents to a religion, others have, until now, grown up hardly giving much thought to God. All, however, have one thing in common—they are on a faith journey. They are on a journey of seeking the priceless treasure of a relationship with God.

The activities in this section are intended to focus on that one thing the people have in common —the faith journey on which they are embarking— and thereby to build community so that the people will experience the process of Christian initiation not as a random collectivity of individuals but as fellow seekers, fellow journeyers who offer one another mutual support along the road.

1.

ACTIVITIES DURING THE TIME OF INQUIRY

Early in the Inquiry sessions, all participants should be encouraged to tell the stories of their religious pilgrimage thus far. The activities in this section will begin the process of community building among the candidates, leaders and sponsors. The religious journey of a group is smoother and quicker when everyone knows something about each other's religious pilgrimage.

People may feel uneasy at first about sharing their personal stories. However, often the participants will find that they have more in common than they suspected. They will be encouraged by hearing the struggles and difficulties others have experienced and will see how God has been active and present in the most unlikely situations. Leaders may want to call upon a sponsor to share his or her experience first in order to break the ice. Whereas sharing ideas can sometimes distance people—because they tend to defend their own ideas and try to persuade others to adopt them—sharing experiences tends to bring people together. Shared experience creates a strong and immediate bond, because people can easily identify with what others have gone through in similar situations.

The following six activities will also help each participant become more conscious of God's activity in his or her own life and to see how he or she has been led to join this particular group.

Religious Lifeline

PURPOSE

To help participants see that they all have had ups and downs in their faith journeys.

MATERIALS NEEDED

- One pencil for each participant
- One sheet of paper for each participant

DIRECTIONS

Ask the participants to draw across their sheets of paper a straight line representing their life span. At the right end of the line they write the present date, and at the left end they write the approximate date when they first remember being concerned about God. Instruct them to chart the highs and lows of their relationship to God, indicating times when they felt God was close to them and active in their lives (peaks) as well as times when God seemed far away (valleys). At each of the high or low points they should write in a date, the incident, and the people involved.

After everyone has finished, invite each participant to hold up the sheet of paper for all to see and share the high and low points of his or her relationship to God with the entire group. Have the candidates tell why at this time they think God is calling them to take another step in their faith journeys.

When everyone has spoken, point out some experiences that many people in the group have shared. Suggest that the initiation process is a journey they are taking as a group.

A sample lifeline might look something like the one on the next page.

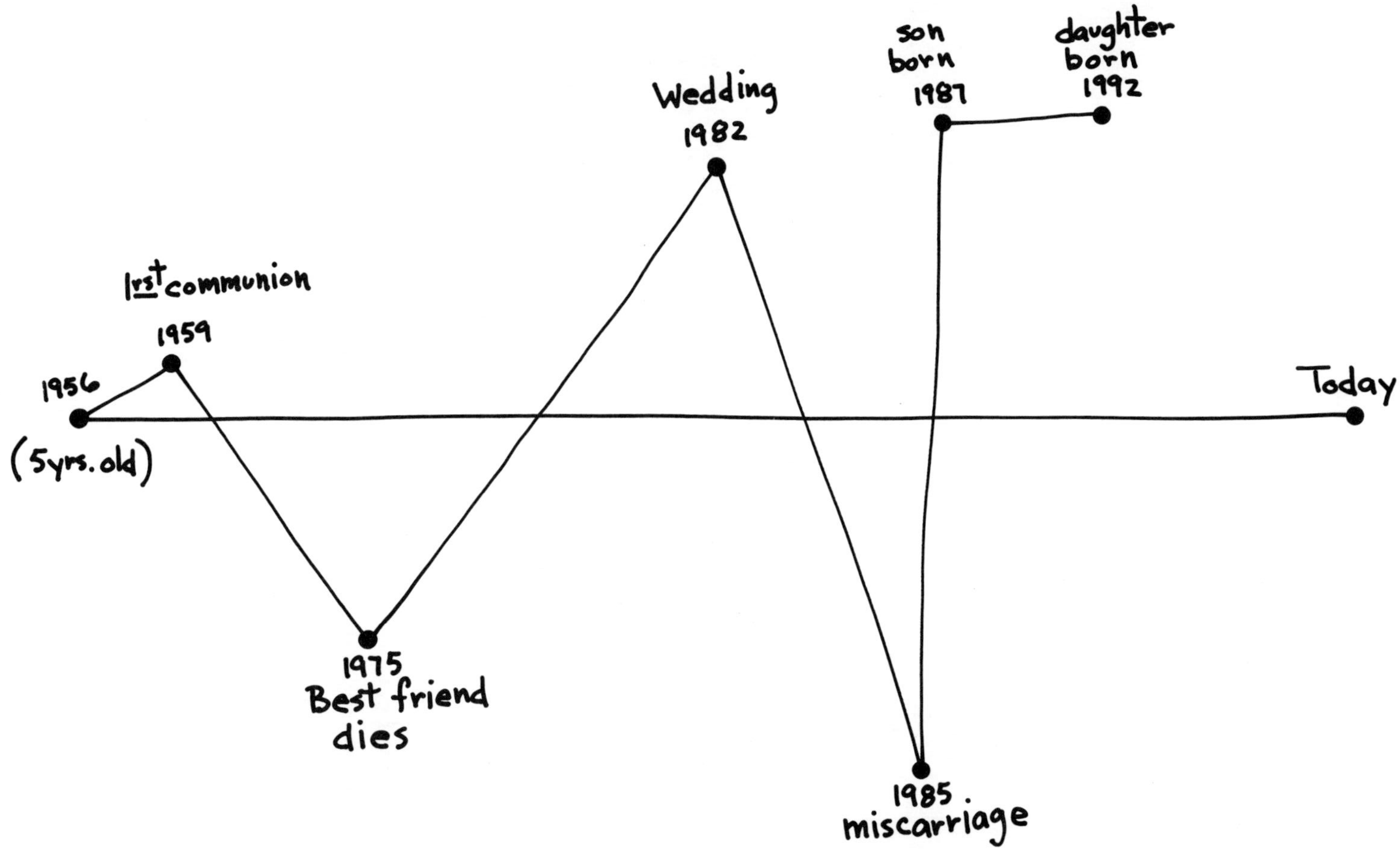
1st communion
1959
1956
(5yrs. old)
1975
Best friend
dies
Wedding
1982
1985
miscarriage
son
born
1987
daughter
born
1992
Today

Religious Topographical Map

PURPOSE

To help participants get in touch with their faith experiences in a "right-brain" way.

MATERIALS NEEDED

- A supply of different colored pencils, pens or markers
- One sheet of paper for each participant

DIRECTIONS

Invite each person to draw a "topographical map" of his or her spiritual history. Various aspects of that landscape can be represented by such map features as mountains, deserts, rivers, swamps, etc. (For example, mountains can be indicated by peaks, rough roads by wiggly lines, detours by road signs, and so forth.) The maps need not be very artistic—this is not a class in cartography!

After everyone is finished, invite the participants to hold up their maps and ask the group to identify the various areas depicted. As a member of the group identifies an area such as a river or swamp, the presenter tells what it stands for. For example: "That is a swamp." "Yes, that was the time I was mired in doubt."

When everyone has finished describing his or her map, ask the participants to identify which other map resonated most with their own experiences. Point out some experiences that many people in the group have shared. Suggest one or two topographical features the entire group could add to their maps to indicate where the group is (at the beginning of a road, for example) or where it is going (over the rainbow).

A sample map might look like the one on the next page.

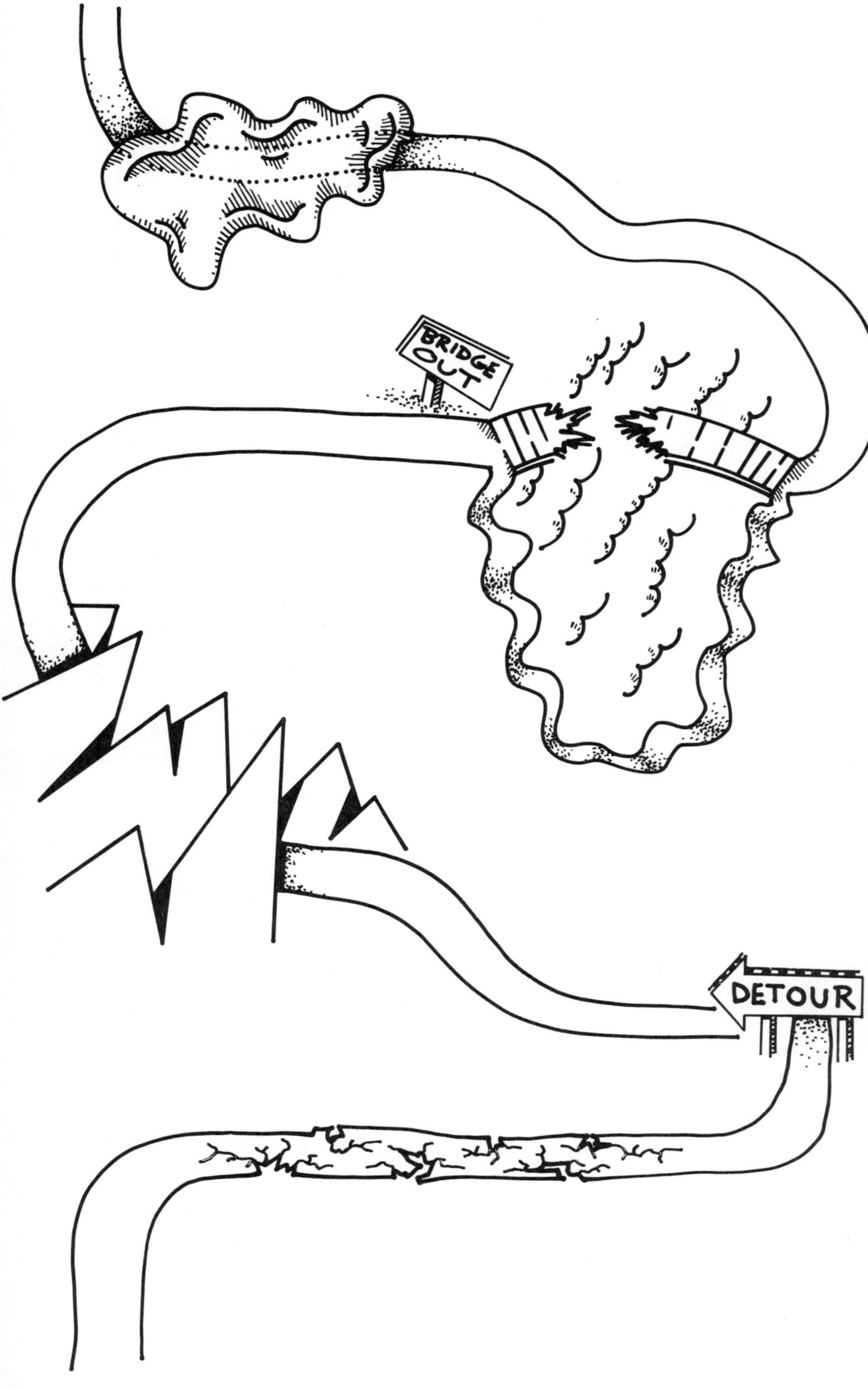
BRIDGE
OUT
DETOUR

Creating a Story

PURPOSE

To have participants use their imagination to describe their religious experiences.

MATERIALS NEEDED

- One pencil for each participant
- One sheet of paper for each participant

DIRECTIONS

Ask each participant to create a fairy tale, a story about animals or a story set on some distant planet which recounts the adventures and misadventures on their religious journey. They must tell the story in the third person and not use the personal pronouns "I," "me" or "my." Give them a few minutes to think about a story line and to write down an outline. When everyone is ready invite the participants to share their stories in small groups.

Someone's story might go like this: Once upon a time in a far-off land, a young man set out to find a hidden treasure that he had heard about. At first people were helpful, guiding him along the right road, but soon different people were giving him different directions. He was so confused he decided to give up looking for the treasure and settle down. He started a business, got married, and had children, but still he wondered where the treasure was. Some of his friends said there was no treasure; others suggested various places it might be. His wife always smiled when he asked her, but she never told him which way to go. One day he realized that she had found the treasure and had had it all along. He asked her to share it with him, and she invited him to join her in church.

If there is time, have each small group choose one person to repeat his or her story for the entire group. When they have finished, ask what insights or conclusions about common threads in the participants' faith journeys people have come to based on hearing these stories. Have the group try to come up with a theme for a happy ending that would fit all the stories told.

Creating a Collage

PURPOSE

To emphasize the similarity between various participants' religious or spiritual *experiences.*

MATERIALS NEEDED

- Lots of old magazines with pictures
- Several pairs of scissors
- One large poster board
- Tape

DIRECTIONS

Have a pile of magazines available for the group members to search through during the session. Ask them to cut out at most three or four pictures that in some way represent important events, positive or negative, on their faith journeys. (If time is short, have participants complete this step prior to the session.)

Invite each person to display his or her pictures to the entire group and explain how each picture symbolizes a spiritual or religious experience of his or her faith journey. After all have shared their pictures, ask the group to identify similarities in the positive or negative experiences they have had and their religious or spiritual significance. Then tape all the pictures on the poster board to create a group collage of experiences. Discuss a few things the group might do together to create a shared religious or spiritual experience.

Recounting the Call

PURPOSE

To identify the event or person that/who moved each participant to join the initiation program and to summarize what participants hope to achieve.

MATERIALS NEEDED

- One pencil for each participant
- Activity Sheet A, one copy for each participant, copied front to back (see pp. 123–24)

DIRECTIONS

Introduce this activity with the following or similar words:

> Our journey to God moves at an uneven pace. There are times when the Divine feels close and times when it feels far away or even totally absent. Christians believe, however, that God is always with us—calling us, inviting us through the people and events of our lives. This call is often loudest when we feel that something is missing in our lives or when tragedy strikes. Some people hear the call most clearly when beauty or some happy moment gives them a glimpse of the Something More, of that which is Beyond. In any case, it is helpful to recall the course of our religious journey and identify how God has been leading us to our present state.

Have each participant fill out Activity Sheet A. Read the directions aloud and make sure everyone understands what is to be done. Allow sufficient time for all to finish the entire exercise.

Then invite the participants to form small groups and share their answers. Finally, call the people back to the large group to share a summary (not a verbatim report) of how the people in the small groups answered the four questions. Have the participants agree on composites to the answers to questions three and four and offer it to the group as a unified statement of purpose for the initiation program. (Perhaps even vote to adopt it as a formal statement.)

My Ideas about Church

PURPOSE

To bring to mind and express the participants' *ideas* about church.

MATERIALS NEEDED

- One pencil for each participant
- Activity Sheet B, one copy for each participant, copied on two separate sheets (see pp. 125–26)

DIRECTIONS

Introduce this activity with these or similar words:

> This activity has two purposes. One is to help each of us become clear about his or her ideas of what a church is and should be. At this point in the initiation process we need to begin to see how these ideas are the same as, similar to, or different from the Catholic view of church. The second purpose is to bring to surface any questions you have about the Catholic Church. It is necessary to answer your questions about the church before we can move on to a presentation of what the church says and does.

Have each participant fill out Activity Sheet B. Read the directions aloud and make sure everyone understands what is to be done. Allow sufficient time for all to finish the entire exercise.

Here are two suggested ways of proceeding with the activity:

Either: invite the people to form small groups in which to share their answers. (The "ones" and the "fives" ought to spark a lively discussion!)

Or: taking one statement at a time, ask the entire group and tabulate all the responses. This will give the group members (as well as the leaders) a sense of how the people in the group think about church.

Reminder: In neither case should there be any "correcting" of answers by others in the group!

While the discussion takes place, one of the leaders should collect the participants' questions about the church and combine those that are similar. If there is time, answer those you can and answer the remaining questions later, either in the group or individually, as appropriate.

2.

ACTIVITIES AT THE TIME OF ACCEPTANCE INTO THE ORDER OF CATECHUMENS

Those who are accepted as catechumens are already considered "members" of the church. Membership in the church is a relationship with mutual responsibilities and benefits. At this stage the catechumen acknowledges, "Yes, I want to continue the process of becoming a full member of the church." The community, in turn, assures them, "We want you to continue the process of becoming a full member of our church, and we will help you to become one." The people who principally carry out this pledge of the community are the leaders and facilitators of the initiation program, the sponsors and other companions, and the other candidates.

The two activities in this section help all the people in the group express their commitment to make the journey of faith together. They give the candidates an opportunity to ask for the help they need from the group and its individual members and to promise the help that they will offer in turn to the group and to each member.

Come, Follow Me

PURPOSE

To elicit a commitment from each of the participants to help each other during and after this program.

MATERIALS NEEDED

- Marker and tape
- A large, long piece of newsprint posted on a wall, with a large *Chi Rho* drawn in a bright color at its right end
- Bible

DIRECTIONS

Read aloud Mark 1:14–22, "Come after me!"

Invite a discussion by the entire group on the following questions:

What in the message and life of Jesus is causing you to want to follow him?

To follow Jesus what kind of help do you need from this group?

How do you think you can contribute to this group?

This is a good opportunity to bring out the importance of the following contributions:

- being present for each session
- sharing honestly
- listening to others and accepting what they say
- supporting the others in the group.

(If one or more of these points is not mentioned, the leaders may wish gently to suggest them, in words such as: "I have also found that [e.g., sharing honestly] helps a group run smoothly.")

At the end of the discussion, invite each person to go to the newsprint and make a stick drawing of himself or herself with a heavy marker. As they do this, each person is to name what he or she will contribute to the group to help the others. The first person draws his or her figure so that it is attached to the *Chi Rho*. The second person attaches his or her drawing to that of the first person and so on, until a long line of people are following Jesus. Ask the group what the entire drawing suggests about the enrollment of the candidates in the order of catechumens.

The results may look something like this:

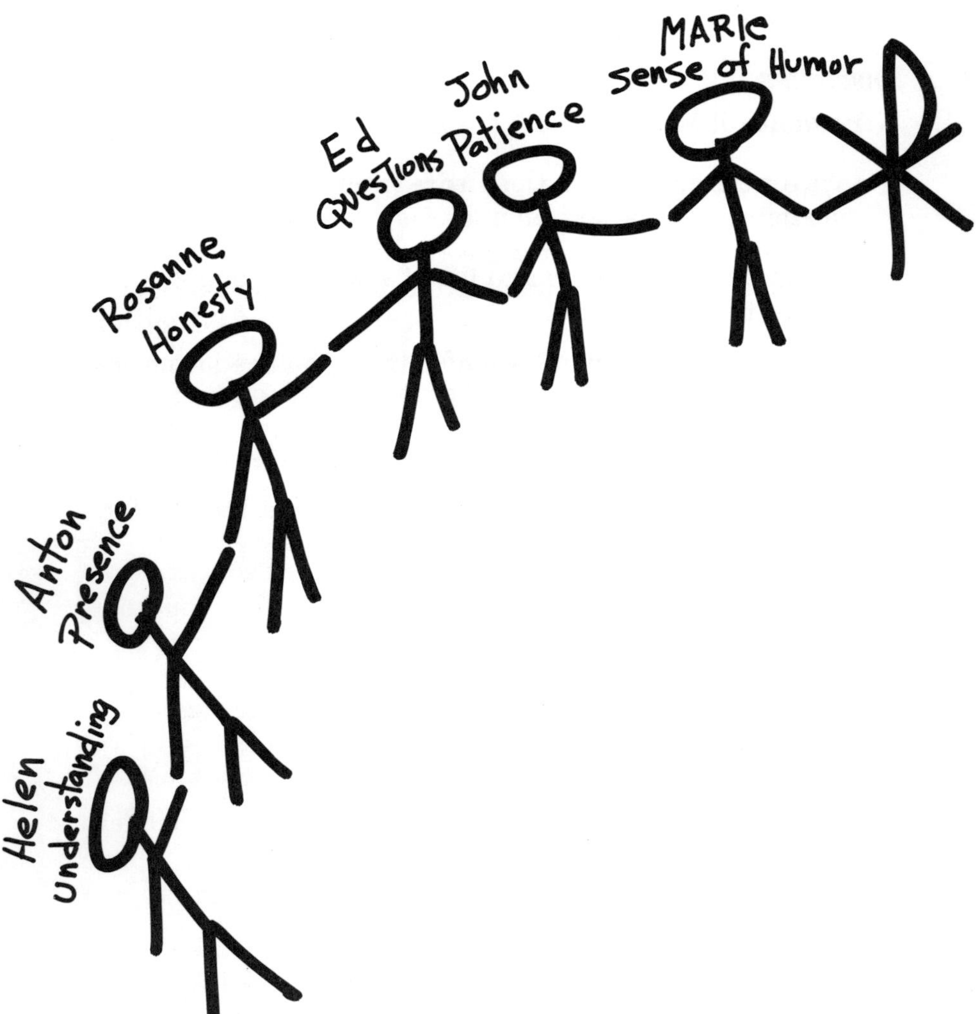

We All Need One Another

PURPOSE

To show how important every part is to the success of the whole.

MATERIALS NEEDED

- Activity Sheet C, one copy for each participant (see p.127)
- Newsprint or chalkboard, on which someone has drawn a large outline of a car
- Marker and tape or chalk

DIRECTIONS

Introduce the activity with these or similar words:

> As the candidates are accepted into the Order of Catechumens, we all embark on a journey together. Our group here is the vehicle—or car—in which we will make that journey. Think of yourself as one part of that car, a part without which the car would not operate or would not run smoothly. There are thousands of parts on a car, some big, some very small, but all contribute to making a ride in the car enjoyable and trouble-free. Some of these parts are absolutely necessary, such as the wheels. Others are decoration, like hood ornaments. Some are large, such as the engine. Others are small, such as the nuts that hold the wheel on. Each part, however, makes a contribution to the whole. Think about which part of the car you want to be (symbolically) on this journey and what your part will contribute to the success of the journey.

Have each participant fill out Activity Sheet C. Read the directions aloud and make sure everyone understands what is to be done. Allow sufficient time for all to finish the entire exercise.

Then ask everyone to sit in a circle and, one by one, tell which part of the car they are, why, and what that part will contribute to the success of the group's journey. (It may be advisable for the leader to speak first to give an example of how the activity is to be done.)

After all have spoken, invite a discussion on the following questions:

> A car needs regular maintenance to run smoothly and safely. What are some of the things that need to be done routinely to keep a car in good running condition? Likewise, what are the things we can each do for one another to make our journey run smoothly?

(This may be a good time to emphasize the importance of being present at each session, sharing honestly, accepting and listening to others, and supporting one another. If no one mentions these things, you may wish gently to suggest, for example, "I have found that [e.g., sharing honestly] helps a journey like ours run smoothly.")

> A car can meet obstacles on the road that make the journey difficult. What would be some of the obstacles this group might encounter? How might we overcome them?

(This may be a good opportunity to remind the group that correcting one another, arguing over "correct" answers, and lecturing on the right or wrong way of doing something are discouraged. If any of these things is not mentioned, and especially if you have noticed tendencies toward one or more of them in the group, you can suggest, "I have found that [e.g., correcting one another] can be a big obstacle on a journey such as ours.")

When the discussion has finished, ask each person to go to the chalkboard or newsprint and draw in the appropriate place the part of the car he or she would like to be. Each one should put his or her initial next to that part. Explain that this action symbolizes a pledge to the group to help the sessions run smoothly and efficiently.

3.

ACTIVITIES AT THE TIME OF ELECTION OR ENROLLMENT OF NAMES

The Rite of Election is public testimony to the fitness of the candidates to become members of the church. The community "elects" or chooses those whom it recognizes as having been called by God and gives public testimony that they are worthy to join the church. The candidates are presented to the community and their names inscribed in the Book of the Elect, and the candidates pledge that they will be faithful members of the church.

At the sessions before this liturgical rite is celebrated in church, it is good to have the members of the group accept and affirm each other as worthy to be chosen by the community and enrolled in the Book of the Elect.

Introduce one of three activities that follow with these or similar words:

> We have been together for _____ (weeks/months), and during this time we have witnessed the sincerity of the members of our group and have experienced their help and support. Before celebrating the Rite of Election, let us review our journey together so far.

Then invite each candidate in turn to tell the group how the journey has gone for him or her so far.

When all have spoken, proceed with one of the following activities.

A Bouquet for Ourselves

PURPOSE

To make each participant feel good about himself or herself.

MATERIALS NEEDED

- Two vases, one empty and one filled with fresh cut flowers (one flower for each participant of the group)

DIRECTIONS

Have the participants sit in a circle, with the empty vase on a small table in the middle of the group and the vase with the flowers off to one side. Continue with words to the following effect:

> Bouquets are a time-honored way of saying thanks and affirming people. On the side table are some cut flowers to make a bouquet for our group. One at a time, each participant will pick up a flower, bring it to the vase here in the middle of our circle and express in his or her own words what the group as a whole has meant to him or her.

When all are finished, continue with these or similar words:

> Each of us has chosen to make this journey together. When we did so, we also undertook to help the other members of the group in various ways. Take a moment or two and recall how various members of the group have helped you and/or the group during the past (weeks/months). Then those who wish may share with the group how one person has been a help to him or her.

(During this phase of the activity it is important to ensure that each one of the catechumens is mentioned by name and given a pat on the back for some contribution to the group.)

Beginning to Bloom

PURPOSE

To recognize that the group as a whole and each participant is helpful to each person in the group.

MATERIALS NEEDED

- Sticks, about 4 inches long with a flag or flower cut out of paper pasted on each (one for each participant)
- One pencil for each participant
- One large flower pot with soil in it
- Bible

DIRECTIONS

Read aloud Mark 4:1–20, "Good soil and a bountiful harvest."

Then invite a discussion on the following questions:

In what ways does this group represent good soil that nourishes each of us?

How do you see individual people in the group as good soil helping you give a good yield?

What harvests do we hope to reap?

When you have finished the discussion, give each person one of the little flags or flowers. Ask everyone to write on it one way in which the group is helping him or her to grow. Then one at a time have people place their sticks into the soil in the flower pot and tell what they wrote on them.

Old and New Wine Skins

PURPOSE

To encourage the participants to be open to change and new ideas.

MATERIALS NEEDED

- Activity Sheet D, one copy for each participant (see p. 129)
- A wastebasket
- Bible

DIRECTIONS

Read aloud Mark 2:18–22, "New wine in old wine skins."

Continue with these or similar words:

> Old wine skins lost their flexibility as they aged. New skins were flexible and could expand. With our modern methods of pre-shrunk cloth, we are not too familiar with what happens when an unshrunk piece of cloth is used to repair a garment that has been washed several times. It tears loose and makes the rip worse.
>
> The bridal metaphor in the reading expresses a new relationship established by Jesus between God and God's people. A new way of living and relating to God was revealed. Any attempt, for example, to attach the new discipleship of Jesus to the old practices of the Pharisees will not work. So, too, in baptism a new life needs to be undertaken. We cannot just attach a few new practices to our old way of thinking, our old attitudes, or our old behavior. We are called to change our ideas, our attitudes, and our way of behaving. We are called to put the new wine into new wine skins.

Have each participant fill out Activity Sheet D. Read the directions aloud and make sure everyone understands what is to be done. Allow sufficient time for all to finish the entire exercise.

Then ask those who wish to share with the entire group what they have written. After all have finished sharing, have them tear their papers in two, shred the old wineskin into small pieces, and discard the pieces into the wastebasket. Invite the people to congratulate one another with the kiss of peace.

4.

ACTIVITY AT THE TIME OF SCRUTINIES

The period of Lent is a time of intense spiritual formation. The elect are called to deeper reflection intended to purify their minds and hearts before the Easter sacraments. The Scrutinies are rites meant to heal all that is weak or sinful in the hearts of the elect.

This activity is intended to help participants progress in a genuine deepening of self knowledge and repentance and strengthen their commitment to Christ. It will help them get in touch with their struggles and weaknesses in committing their lives to the Lord. This is especially an opportunity for candidates to express their difficulties to the group and for the group to offer a prayer that they may be strengthened in their final preparation for the sacraments of initiation.

The Struggle to Follow the Lord

PURPOSE

To identify the difficulties participants might be having at this stage in the initiation program.

MATERIALS NEEDED

- One small ball of clay for each participant
- Cassette recorder and cassette tape of reflective music (preferably an instrumental piece)
- Table
- Bible

DIRECTIONS

Ask the participants to sit in one circle around the table. Introduce the activity with the following or similar words:

> As our candidates draw nearer to our full initiation into the church at Easter, it is important to recognize the need for God's continued help and healing in our lives. Everyone struggles with weakness, doubt and sin. If these are left unchecked, they prevent us from fully following the Lord. This activity will help all of us to recognize and name our struggles so that we can bring them to the Lord for the Lord's help and healing. Part of this healing will come from the prayers and support of those in this group and from those in the larger church who struggle with us in our efforts to deepen our relationship with the Lord.
>
> There is a story about Jesus that illustrates perfectly the course of this struggle. Let's listen to the story and see how it sheds light on the struggle we all face.

Read aloud Mark 8:22–26, "A blind man receives his sight."

Discuss the following questions:

> In what way do you see this story as symbolic of your own struggle to see clearly what following Jesus entails?

Jesus had to touch the man's eyes not once but twice. What does this suggest to you about the struggles we face?

Give the participants each a ball of clay and ask them to shape it into a symbol of an issue they are now struggling with. Allow a few minutes, and then invite the participants to share their clay figures with the entire group and explain their significance. After each has shared, have them put their clay symbols on the table in the center of the group.

During the next part of the activity, ask the group to remain silent. While suitable background music is played, invite one of the participants to take all of the individual symbols and mold them into one large ball of clay. When this has been done, ask the person to pass the ball of clay to the person on his or her right. Ask that person to shape the clay into an image that symbolizes a prayer for the struggles he or she has heard expressed in the group. This person then passes the symbol to the person on the right, and that person can improve the figure or make a completely new one. The clay continues to be passed to the right, and each participant can modify or reshape it. If a person is satisfied with the shape, he or she can pass it on without changing it. The clay continues to go around the group until no one makes any more changes in it. The ball of clay may go around the group several times before all are satisfied.

Turn off the music and invite each person to share what he or she tried to express through the clay.

Finally, ask the group to join hands as a sign that they will pray for one another in the final weeks of preparation for the candidates' initiation at Easter. Together, pray the Lord's Prayer.

5.

ACTIVITY AT THE TIME OF BAPTISM

Some of the people in the program may not be preparing for Baptism. They may be preparing to be reconciled with the church community after having been away for a time, and they may or may not share in some of the initiation ceremonies. However, every participant will be leaving behind an old way of life and embracing a new one. At a session before Baptism, it is helpful to place the emphasis on that fact.

This activity is designed to use the baptismal symbol of water in a way that dramatizes change and purification.

Change and Transformation

PURPOSE

To emphasize that the end result of the initiation process should be a radical change of life.

MATERIALS NEEDED

- Black ink in a bottle
- Liquid bleach in a bottle
- One bowl of water
- One dropper
- Bible

DIRECTIONS

Have all the participants sit in a circle around a table. Place the appropriate materials on the table; the bottle of ink should be labeled "old life," and the bottle of bleach should be labeled "new life."

Read aloud Colossians 3:1–17, "Put away the old, put on the new."

Introduce the activity with the following or similar words:

> Most likely, we can honestly say that we have tried to put away the old self and the things that Paul tells us to lay aside. In a very real sense, being baptized [being reconciled, making a profession of faith] is a taking-off of something old and a putting-on of something new.
>
> The process of dying in order to have new life will go on in many ways until we eventually leave this life behind and enter the eternal life that God has in store for us. Each of us at one time or another has had part of us "die" for the sake of something new. Reflect for a few moments on a time in your life when you have made a change, large or small, that required you to leave behind certain things and to take up new ways of being—for example, leaving home to go to school or to be married or to go out on your

own; changing a job; experiencing the death of a loved one; or undergoing a serious physical change.

Recall how you felt: the fears, the anticipation, maybe even the anger or uncertainty. Identify how you feel now about that change, about the things you left behind, and about the new life you have.

Ask each person to share their recollection briefly. Then have the members of the group think of things they are leaving behind—both good and bad—as they become full members of the church. Invite everyone to stand around the table and have each person take a drop of the "old life" and put it into the bowl of water. As the participants do so they may, if they wish, express what they are leaving behind. (Assure them, however, that it is not necessary to say anything.)

When everyone has finished, take the bottle labeled "new life" and say:

This bowl has collected all of our old lives, all of the things from which we have turned away. These things have colored the pure water of the life God wishes for each of us. We now pour this new life of Baptism into the bowl and pray that God will purify each of us once again.

Pour the bleach in the water and wait for the water to clear. Have everyone give each other the kiss of peace and then return to their seats. If there is time, discuss the following questions with the group:

What does this experiment say to you about what we will be doing [at the Easter Vigil, next Sunday]?

How do you feel about the new life which is being given to you and which you are intent upon living?

How would you like this group to help in your continuing efforts to live the life Jesus gives us in Baptism?

6.

ACTIVITY AT THE TIME OF COMMISSIONING

At the last session of the initiation process, it is most helpful to have all the participants review what has occurred on their journey together. The following activity allows participants to articulate the gifts they have received from each other and their commitment to sharing these gifts with others.

Go Forth and Share

Purpose

To affirm the gifts each participant has given and received.

Materials needed

- One colored pen or pencil for each participant
- Sticky labels (enough so that each participant has one for every other member of the group)
- One cross to pin or hang on each participant
- Refreshments

Directions

Introduce the activity with these or similar words:

> We have come on a long journey together and have grown in many ways. As with any journey, there have been high and low points. There may have been times when we wanted to give up and turn back, or times when we felt like stopping along the side of the road. It may have been hard to continue pressing on rather than yield to these detours. But as we traveled, we discovered new things about ourselves, about our relationship with God, and about the people in this group. It is important that we appreciate the progress we have made and see more clearly how each person in the group has helped us. Equally, it is important for us to see how much we meant to others in the group. However, this is not the conclusion of our journey. In a very real sense it is the beginning of a new journey. And so we will conclude with a commissioning ceremony.

Ask the participants to close their eyes and recall their journey together as you briefly review the liturgical rites, the material covered and any important events that happened during the initiation process. An outline of what you wish to say would be helpful to ensure that you are brief and do not leave anything out.

After the review of the journey has been completed, conduct a short commissioning ceremony. Introduce the ceremony with these or similar words:

> An important part of the journey was the support and encouragement we received from others in the group. As Saint Paul has said, "To each individual the manifestation of the Spirit has been given for the benefit of all." (1 Cor. 12:7). When we share ourselves we help others to meet their needs and to grow. It is important that we recognize the help and support we have received from the others in the group.

Then ask the members of the group to think about every other person in the group, about a quality that they have come to admire in that person and which has been helpful to them in their journey. Ask them to make a tag for each person, writing that person's name and quality on it.

When everyone has made a tag for every other person, ask each participant, one at a time, to sit on a chair in the center of the group. Have the group stand around that person and, one at a time, come up, express the quality they admire and attach the tag to the person. After everyone has put a tag on the person, the entire group lays hands on the person and the leader puts a cross on the person, saying: "Go forth and share the Good News of Jesus Christ with others."

When all have been affirmed and commissioned, invite the entire group to share the kiss of peace and to enjoy the refreshments.

SECTION II

Activities to Introduce Specific Areas of Instruction

During the period of catechesis in the initiation process, several major areas of Catholic belief are treated. The following activities are meant to be opening exercises for specific areas of instruction. The purpose of these activities is to allow participants to express their ideas, feelings and questions about the individual area to be covered. Some of these activities call upon the "right side" of the brain, requiring people to use their creative imagination and to look at an idea in a non-verbal way.

The activities also offer the leaders an opportunity to gauge where people are in their thinking about the subject to be presented. People who embark upon the journey of Christian initiation do not come with minds that are completely blank about the doctrines of the Catholic faith. Some have had a Catholic background; others were fervent members of another denomination or faith. Some are lukewarm believers in God; still others have been unchurched or unbelievers all their lives. All come with imperfect knowledge, with prejudices, and especially with questions.

Questions, when expressed and answered, can be of great help in comprehending what is being taught. If they are not asked or answered, however, they can block out much of what is being presented during the initiation process, because the person is always trying to relate the material being presented to that question. Thus it is helpful to allow questions about the material at hand to surface at the beginning of each topic and to answer them as well as possible at that time. This will help clear the way for explaining the core beliefs of Catholicism on each of these important issues.

1.

ACTIVITIES ABOUT GOD

One of the great challenges in spiritual growth is purifying one's concept of God. People carry with them many different images of God—from the harsh, vengeful judge to the "Santa Claus" God who gives them whatever they ask for. They do not realize that every new image of God needs to be questioned or refined. It is important to discover what people's experience of God has been and how they think and feel about the Divinity.

Each of the following four activities focuses on either people's *experiences, ideas* or *feelings* about God. However, the discussion of the activity can and should easily lead into all aspects of participants' relationship to God.

Signs of God

PURPOSE

To encourage participants to become aware of how they imagine God.

MATERIALS NEEDED

- Table on which are four or five times as many items as there are people in the group—items such as flowers, rocks, stuffed animals, books, food items, small tools or kitchen appliances, pieces of string or rope or paper
- Bible

DIRECTIONS

Introduce the activity with these or similar words:

> The Hebrew people of the Old Testament saw God acting through very visible signs or symbols. One such symbol was manifest during the exodus from Egypt.

Read aloud Exodus 13:17–18, 21–22, "The Lord preceded them."

Then continue:

> For the Hebrews the pillars of cloud and fire were symbols of God's protective care as they ventured out of Egypt toward the Promised Land.

Ask the participants to look at the items on the table in silence. Invite each person to pick one item that speaks to him or her about God's ongoing presence in his or her life. When everyone has chosen an item, invite each person to tell the entire group why this particular item is a sign or symbol of God's ongoing presence in his or her life.

My Experience of God

PURPOSE

To help participants recall or share their various *experiences* of God.

MATERIALS NEEDED

- Chalkboard or newsprint
- Chalk or marker

DIRECTIONS

On the board or newsprint have the following pairs printed:

Light / Dark

Warm / Cold

Sun / Moon

Calm / Wind

Near / Far

Rain / Drought

Sunny / Cloudy

Ask the participants to look at the list of pairs and select two or three pairs in which they have experienced both extremes in their relationship with God. Then invite them to share their experiences in small groups. (For example, God might have been experienced as both strong and weak, trustworthy and unreliable, etc.)

Finally, call the entire group together and list the various characteristics of God suggested by the different experiences they have mentioned in their small groups.

My Feelings about God

Purpose

To enable participants to express their *feelings* about God.

Materials needed

- A selection of as many different 12-inch pieces of colored yarn as you can collect—several pieces of each color and a wide range of colors

Directions

Introduce the activity in these or similar words:

> Colors can symbolize or signify different things. For example, green can mean inexperienced, envious, environmentally correct or, on a traffic light, indicate "go." Yellow can symbolize cowardice or indicate "caution." Blue may mean "sad" or also "loyal."
>
> Many people cannot put a specific name on their feelings about God, but they might be able to choose a color or two that captures their feelings. This exercise is about how you feel, not about how you think.

Ask the participants to pick two pieces of yarn, one color to express how they feel about God at this time in their lives and one to express how they felt about God at some other time in their lives. Then invite them to hold up the two pieces of yarn and try to explain to the large group their reasons for selecting them. (They may not be able to explain. It might just be a "feeling," and that's O.K.)

Finally, have people tie the strings together in one long string and lay the string on the ground surrounding the entire group. Then say the Lord's Prayer or a spontaneous prayer together.

My Ideas about God

PURPOSE

To surface the *thoughts* and *ideas* the participants have about God.

MATERIALS NEEDED

- One pencil for each participant
- Activity Sheet E, one copy for each participant, copied on two separate sheets (see pp. 131–32)

DIRECTIONS

Have each participant fill out Activity Sheet E. Read the directions aloud and make sure everyone understands what is to be done. Allow sufficient time for all to finish the entire exercise.

Then invite participants to share their answers in small groups and describe what in their lives (events or people, for example) has caused them to answer as they did.

Having allowed sufficient time for this, gather the small groups together and ask the entire group what attitudes or feelings toward God would these different ideas of God generate.

While the discussion takes place, one of the leaders should collect the participants' questions about God and combine those that are similar. If there is time, answer those questions you can and answer the remaining questions later, either in the group or individually, as appropriate.

2.

ACTIVITIES ABOUT THE OLD TESTAMENT

Before beginning to learn about the Catholic faith, people need a sense that the present has its roots in the past. The process of Christian initiation is designed to bring people to know and love the Lord. To do this, they need to understand that Jesus did not just pop into history from outer space. He was born at a particular time, in a particular culture and to a particular family. Jesus was a Jew of the first century. He came from a small hill town that existed outside the mainstream of his society. Nevertheless, he came from a people who were strong in their Jewish beliefs and practices. He was a good Jew who knew and loved his heritage. The Old Testament or the Hebrew Bible tells the story of Jesus' people. To understand him, we need to understand that story.

The following four activities focus on the Old Testament and will help participants recognize its importance. In the process, leaders will get an idea of the level of the participants' knowledge of the Bible.

Flow of Consciousness

PURPOSE

To help participants articulate what they think and feel about the Old Testament.

MATERIALS NEEDED

- One piece of paper for each participant
- Chalkboard or newsprint
- Chalk or marker

DIRECTIONS

Tell the group that you are going to give them a list of words, one at a time. As soon as they hear a word they are to write down whatever comes into their minds. They are not to censor the words or give "correct" or "pious" responses. They are to write whatever comes immediately to mind.

In choosing the list of words that you will use in this exercise, be sure to include the words "Bible" and "Old Testament" and to intersperse "everyday" words with some words related to the Old Testament, such as "prophet," "flood," "ark" and so forth. Following is a sample list of other words you might use:

Law	Prophet	Friend	Summer
Blanket	Yahweh	Covenant	Flood
Ark	Hot dog	Ford	Home
Roller coaster	Creation	Salvation	Exodus

Give the group only a brief moment to write after each word. Stress that they must respond quickly. When finished with the list, ask the participants to read their response to each word, but not to repeat what someone else has expressed. Write the different responses on the board or newsprint. Because this is an introduction to the Old Testament, eliminate the "everyday" words and responses. Then ask what the remaining words and responses suggest about people's ideas about the Old Testament.

Finally, invite a discussion on the following questions:

What has been your experience in reading the Old Testament?

How has it helped you?

What difficulties have you experienced with it?

People of the Old Testament

PURPOSE

To help participants become conscious of what they know about some of the people in the Old Testament.

MATERIALS NEEDED

- Chalkboard or newsprint
- Chalk or marker
- Bible

DIRECTIONS

Introduce the activity by explaining that many characters from the Old Testament are mentioned in the Catholic liturgy. They are our ancestors in the faith who have walked in the same path we are walking. They have laid the foundation for our Christian faith. Therefore, an important question we may ask ourselves is: What can we learn from these people that will help us in our faith journey?

List on the blackboard or newsprint the following names: Adam, Eve, Abraham, Sarah, Jacob, Rebecca, Joseph, Moses, Samuel, David, Solomon, Ruth, Judith, Samson, Job, Isaiah, Jeremiah, Maccabees, Daniel and any other Old Testament figure that you wish. It will not be necessary to talk about each one.

Divide into small groups, and be sure that sponsors or leaders are in each group. Invite participants who wish to do so to pick out their favorite name from the list and tell why that person is important or meaningful to them.

When the small groups have finished, pull the entire group back together and read one or two stories from the Bible about key people in the Old Testament. If there is time, ask the group to discuss what these stories suggest about their own journeys of faith.

The Roots of My Faith

PURPOSE

To help participants recognize the religious traditions that have formed their present beliefs and practices.

MATERIALS NEEDED

- One pencil for each participant
- Activity Sheet F, one copy for each participant, copied front to back (see pp.133–34)

DIRECTIONS

Introduce the activity with words to this effect:

Knowing and understanding the family background of a person helps us to know and appreciate that person better. We will be looking at the Old Testament as the history of the religious family into which Jesus was born and as our own history. Many of our own practices and beliefs have their origins in Judaism. In fact, Christians, Jews, and Muslims claim the same faith ancestors—Abraham, Moses and the prophets.

But each of us also has an individual religious history as well, which often reaches back several generations. The better we understand our own history, the better we will appreciate where we are and how we got there.

Have each participant fill out Activity Sheet F. Read the directions aloud and make sure everyone understands what is to be done. Allow sufficient time for all to finish the entire exercise.

Then ask participants to share their trees in small groups. When they have finished, call the entire group back together and ask what people have learned about their own and others' religious backgrounds. Finally, discuss why it is important to know something of the Old Testament if we are to understand Jesus.

A finished tree might look like the one on the next page.

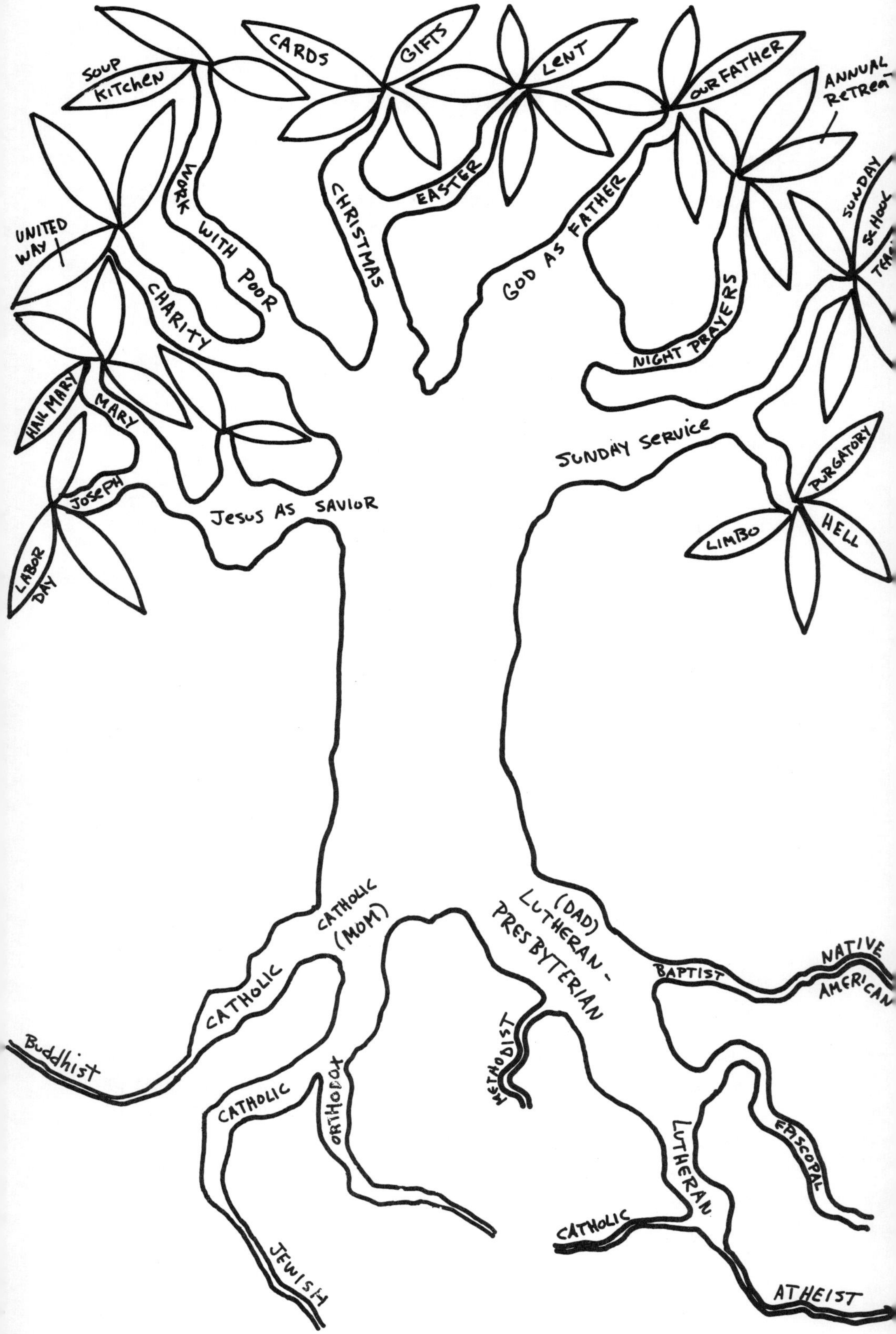
SOUP KITCHEN
CARDS
GIFTS
LENT
OUR FATHER
ANNUAL RETREAT
WORK WITH POOR
CHRISTMAS
EASTER
GOD AS FATHER
SUNDAY SCHOOL
UNITED WAY
CHARITY
NIGHT PRAYERS
HAIL MARY
MARY
SUNDAY SERVICE
PURGATORY
JOSEPH
JESUS AS SAVIOR
LIMBO
HELL
LABOR DAY
CATHOLIC (MOM)
(DAD) LUTHERAN-PRESBYTERIAN
NATIVE AMERICAN
BAPTIST
CATHOLIC
Buddhist
METHODIST
CATHOLIC
ORTHODOX
EPISCOPAL
LUTHERAN
CATHOLIC
JEWISH
ATHEIST

What I Believe about the Bible

PURPOSE

To surface the basic attitudes of the participants toward the Bible.

MATERIALS NEEDED

- One pencil for each participant
- Activity Sheet G, one copy for each participant, copied on two separate sheets (see pp. 135–36)

DIRECTIONS

Have each participant fill out Activity Sheet G. Read the directions aloud and make sure everyone understands what is to be done. Allow sufficient time for all to finish the entire exercise.

Then invite participants to share their answers in small groups. Caution them not to try to correct other people's ideas or to impose their own ideas on others. The purpose of the activity is for each person to become clear on what he or she thinks. In the ensuing sessions, the Catholic approach to the Bible should be explained by the leaders or an outside speaker.

While the discussion takes place, one of the leaders should collect the participants' questions about the Bible and combine those that are similar. If there is time, answer those questions you can and answer the remaining questions later, either in the group or individually, as appropriate.

3.

ACTIVITIES ABOUT JESUS

It would be hard to find someone in our culture who has not heard about Jesus of Nazareth. Most people in the initiation process already have all sorts of questions, ideas, images and feelings about him. Before they can begin to hear the Good News that Jesus came to bring, they need to have their questions about him answered. Otherwise those questions, constantly in the back of their minds, will distract them from paying full attention to the material being presented.

The following four activities have been designed to encourage people to think about and share their ideas and feelings about Jesus and to raise any questions they might have with the group.

How I Came to Know Jesus

PURPOSE

To have participants share their *experience* in getting to know Jesus.

MATERIALS NEEDED

- One pencil for each participant
- Activity Sheet H, one copy for each participant (see p. 137)
- Chalkboard or newsprint
- Chalk or marker

DIRECTIONS

Have each participant fill out Activity Sheet H. Read the directions aloud and make sure everyone understands what is to be done. Allow sufficient time for all to finish the entire exercise.

Then divide participants into small groups and ask them to share their answers with the others in their group. When the small group discussions are finished, reassemble the entire group. List the various ways that people have come to know Jesus. Then point out that all Christians continue to learn about Jesus and that the initiation process is one more way or opportunity to get to know him better.

Symbols of Jesus

PURPOSE

To focus on traditional symbols of Jesus and their meaning for today.

MATERIALS NEEDED

- One pencil for each participant
- One sheet of paper for each participant
- One candle, one loaf of bread, one glass of wine, two Bibles and a small shepherd's crook of wood or paper

DIRECTIONS

Pass the candle, bread, wine, one of the Bibles, and the shepherd's crook around (one at a time) among the entire group one at a time, reading the appropriate Gospel text with each one.

Symbol: Light

Light the candle and read aloud John 1:4–9 and John 9:5. During the reading, pass the candle around among the group.

Symbol: Bread and wine

Read aloud John 6:35, 54–55. During the reading, pass the bread and wine around among the group.

Symbol: Book

Read aloud John 1:1. During the reading, pass the book around among the group.

Symbol: Shepherd's crook

Read aloud John 10:14–15. During the reading, pass the shepherd's crook around among the group.

After all the readings have been completed, ask the entire group to reflect on which symbols, or others, speak to them individually about their relationships with Jesus at this time in their lives. Invite those who wish to share their reflections with the group.

Who Has Jesus Been to Me?

PURPOSE

To help participants see how their image of Jesus has changed over time.

MATERIALS NEEDED

- One pencil for each participant
- One sheet of paper for each participant
- Chalkboard or newsprint
- Chalk or marker

DIRECTIONS

Ask the participants to reflect on the various images they've had of Jesus in their lives: for example, when they were in school and thought of Jesus as a great teacher, or when they were sick and looked at him as a healer, or when were they treated unjustly and used him as a role model. Have them indicate on paper different periods in their lives and how they saw Jesus and related to him at that time. Start by sharing something from your own life as an example.

After allowing sufficient time for the people to write, invite them to share their images of Jesus in small groups and how their relationship to him changed from one period to another.

If there is time, bring everyone back together in a large group and list on the chalkboard or newsprint the various images people have had of Jesus. Discuss which images are helpful or not helpful to individuals in the group.

An example of a completed list might look like the one on the next page.

Elementary School → Big Brother

High School → Best Friend

Marriage → Brother-in-Law

After Car Accident → Healer

When Child died → Consoler

Now → Hero

Who Is Jesus Christ?

PURPOSE

To surface some of the ambiguity in the participants' thinking about the divinity and humanity of Jesus.

MATERIALS NEEDED

- One pencil for each participant
- Activity Sheet I, one copy for each participant, copied on two separate sheets (see pp. 139–40)

DIRECTIONS

Have each participant fill out Activity Sheet I. Read the directions aloud and make sure everyone understands what is to be done. Allow sufficient time for all to finish the entire exercise.

Assure participants that this is not a "test" that will be "corrected." When they have finished, have them share and explain their answers in small groups. Then reassemble in the larger group and ask each group to report which statements caused the most disagreement and why they think this is so.

While the discussion takes place, one of the leaders should collect the participants' questions about Jesus and combine those that are similar. If there is time, answer those questions you can and answer the remaining questions later, either in the group or individually, as appropriate.

4.

ACTIVITIES ABOUT THE CHURCH

More and more people are having less and less experience of church. Some may have had practically no contact with a church. For others a short stay in Sunday school may have been their only contact. Still others may have had a painful or very negative experience of church. In any case, it is important to allow people to express their feelings about church and their expectations of it before treating the question catechetically.

It is important for participants to realize that their experience of this initiation process is also an experience of church and that both the *universal* church and the *local* church are encountered on an ongoing basis in the parish, in its liturgies, and in its activities. The following four activities are designed to help people become conscious of their feelings and expectations of church.

Introduce any of the following activities with these or similar words:

> Each of us has had some experience of church. We may have been to a church service such as a wedding or a funeral, we may be regular churchgoers or we may have stopped going completely at some time or another. In any case, we have feelings about church, ideas about what church is and expectations of church. We will use this activity to express some of these feelings and experiences.

Models of Church

PURPOSE

To show participants that there are many models or ways of thinking about church.

MATERIALS NEEDED

- Building materials such as wooden blocks, Legos, Tinker Toys

DIRECTIONS

Either: form small groups and give each group some of the building materials. Ask the groups each to build a model that expresses what they think church is. (For example, a group might build a circle or a chain or a tower.) Everyone in the group must agree on what is to be built. When they have finished, invite each small group to show their model to the entire large group, so that the others may guess what the model represents. If no one interprets the model correctly, then the group who made it must explain it. If there is time, invite each participant to express what he or she wants from the church.

And/Or: Distribute a sufficient amount of building material to each participant. Ask each person to build something that expresses what he or she wants from church. (For example, someone might make a shield or a loaf of bread or a cross.) When all have finished, invite each person in turn to show his or her model to the large group and to explain its meaning.

Envisioning the Church

PURPOSE

To enable participants to identify symbols of positive and negative experiences of church.

MATERIALS NEEDED

- A supply of magazines with pictures
- One pair of scissors for each participant

DIRECTIONS

Ask each person to select from the magazines two pictures, one to express what they would like church to be in their lives and the second to express how they have actually experienced church. The pictures chosen may not contain people—they must be scenes, animals or inanimate objects. Then invite all the participants in turn to show their pictures to the entire group, and to explain why they chose those particular symbols for church.

Here are examples of two photos people might choose:

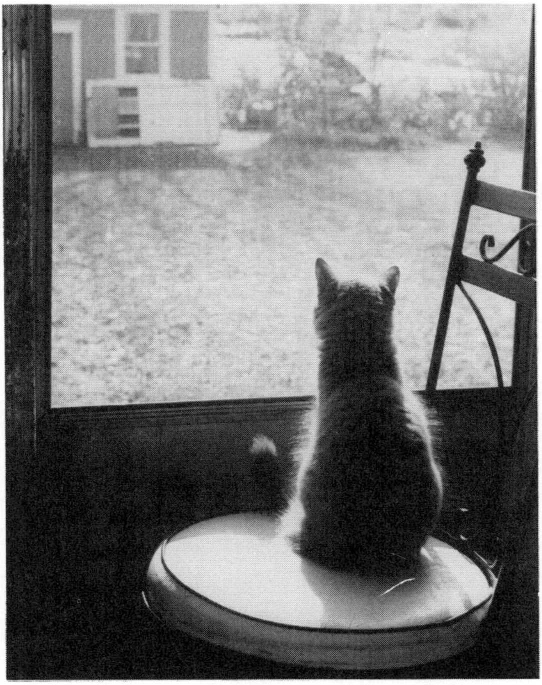

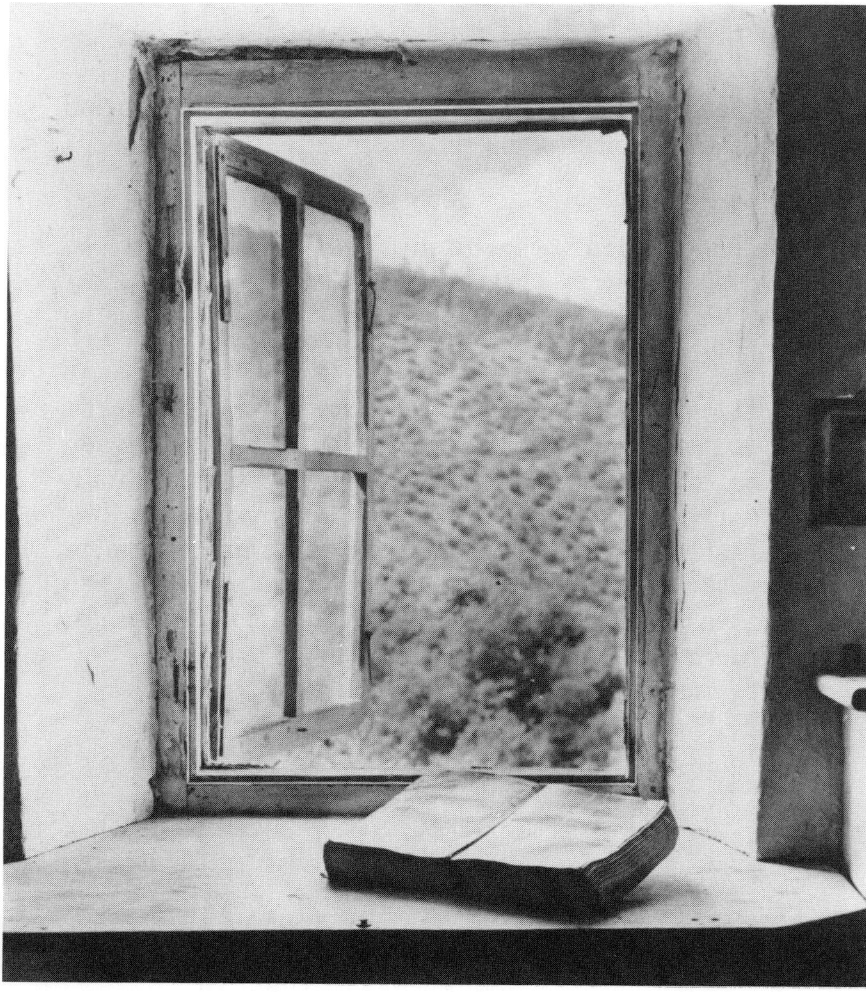

Images of the Church

PURPOSE

To emphasize that the participants' images of the church change over time.

MATERIALS NEEDED

- Pipe cleaners in three different colors (these can be obtained from a craft shop, drug store or teacher's supply store)

DIRECTIONS

Form small groups and ask each person to take several pipe cleaners and form them into a sign or symbol to express each of the following in turn:

- how he or she felt about the church at some low point in life
- how he or she feels about the church at the present time
- what he or she thinks the church is
- what he or she wants from the church.

Then ask each small group to take all of their pipe cleaners and form them into one new symbol of how they as a group feel about the church. When they have done this, invite them to share their symbol with the large group.

The Church Is Like . . .

Purpose

To help participants identify and share their *feelings* about the church.

Materials needed

- Activity Sheet J, one copy for each participant, copied on two separate sheets (see pp. 141–42)
- Chalkboard or newsprint
- Chalk or marker

Directions

Urge participants to relax, forget their theological words and associate the images on the Activity Sheet with their feelings about the church. Before the group begins the activity, explain that there are no right or wrong answers. The purpose of the activity is not to test their *knowledge* about the church but to let them express their *feelings* about the church.

Have each participant fill out Activity Sheet J. Read the directions aloud and make sure everyone understands what is to be done. Allow sufficient time for all to finish the entire exercise.

When all have finished, invite participants to share in their small groups THREE choices that they each made and explain why they made them.

This activity can also be a fine lead-in to a discussion by the entire group of the five models of the church proposed by Fr. Avery Dulles, S.J.* If you wish, you may continue this activity by naming his models on the chalkboard or newsprint:

- community
- institution
- sacrament
- servant
- herald

Then ask how many people chose the following:

(2) station wagon. Explain that it could be considered an image of the church as *community,* because people travel together in it.

(12) pyramid. Explain that it could be considered an image of the church as *institution,* because the base of the pyramid symbolizes baptism, which is the foundation of all church membership, while the top of the pyramid symbolizes the hierarchy of people holding different levels of authority and responsibility.

(13) phone conversation. Explain that it could be considered an image of the church as *sacrament,* because there is dialogue and interchange between God and God's people in the sacraments.

(14) dog. Explain that the dog could be considered an image of the church as *servant,* because dogs care for and serve their masters.

(15) radio station. Explain that this could be considered an image of the church as *herald,* because its purpose is to spread the word.

While the discussion takes place, one of the leaders should collect the participants' questions about the church and combine those that are similar. If there is time, answer those questions you can and answer the remaining questions later, either in the group or individually, as appropriate.

**Models of the Church* (Garden City, NY: Doubleday & Co., 1974)

5.

ACTIVITIES ABOUT THE SACRAMENTS

As Catholics we believe that God acts in our lives through events, people and objects. The seven sacraments are signs of God's activity at critical times in our lives. They are not merely formal rituals that are ends in themselves. Rather, they truly do something to us and for us. For people to begin to appreciate this fact, they first need to appreciate the role of signs and symbols in communication.

The following three activities lead from the impersonal through the personal to the universal and can, if time permits, be done consecutively as one activity. Alternately, you may wish, as usual, to choose the activity or activities that are suitable for your particular group.

Symbols and Signs around Us

Purpose

To help participants become conscious that they are constantly surrounded by all types of signs and symbols.

Materials needed

- None

Directions

Begin with these or similar words:

> We live in a world of symbol and sign. They interpret reality for us. They guide us. They instruct us. In fact, we are surrounded by so many signs and symbols that we often do not recognize them for what they are. For example, the words on a page are signs of an idea or image we have in our mind. But the words themselves are merely ink arranged in a certain arbitrary form. The same idea can be conveyed by many different symbols using the Roman, Arabic or Chinese alphabets.
>
> The difference between signs and symbols is not easy to grasp. A symbol is something that has an *inherent* connection with the idea or thing it signifies. Thus, *water* has an inherent connection with *cleansing*. A sign has no such connection and is merely arbitrary. A *red* light, for example, means *stop* but there is no *inherent* connection between red and danger. It is an arbitrary connection agreed upon by a society.

Invite the participants in the entire group to look around the room and identify any object which they see as a sign or symbol. As people identify an object, they should call it out and tell what it symbolizes to them. Then ask everyone to take one thing from his or her pocket, purse or wallet that is a symbol or sign of who or what he or she is (for example, a set of keys, a credit card, a drivers license, a medical alert band, a picture of loved ones). Invite each person in turn to show his or her object and ask the group to say what the object says about the person and whether it is a symbol or a sign.

When the exercise is finished, discuss with the group why signs and symbols are so necessary in our lives and what would happen in society if people refused to recognize or follow the ones they encounter every day in so many ways.

Signs and Symbols of Love

PURPOSE

To open the imaginations of the participants to the creation of symbols and signs to represent the abstract idea of love.

MATERIALS NEEDED

- One small lump of modeling clay for each participant

DIRECTIONS

Introduce the activity by stating that signs and symbols communicate on a different level than words and often say more than words can. Then ask the participants to use their clay to make a sign or symbol that expresses the love or care someone has shown them. They are not to make a *replica* of something good or beautiful that someone has given them (e.g., a wedding ring). Instead, they are to fashion a new *sign* or *symbol* that shows what the person they have in mind communicated or meant to them. Ask that they not talk while creating their models.

When all have finished, invite each person in turn to share his or her creation with the large group and explain its meaning.

If time permits, ask the participants to reshape the clay into a *sign* or *symbol* through which they themselves express "I love you" to another person. Again, invite each person to share his or her creation with the group.

Finally, ask the participants to form small groups and to put all their pieces of clay together into one lump. Then explain that, without any discussion or speaking, one person is to take the ball of clay and fashion it into a sign or symbol of God's love for us. (They should stretch their imagination and find a symbol other than a heart!) Without speaking, this person then passes the clay to the next person who can accept, refine or reform the clay in any way he or she chooses. This person, again without speaking, passes it on to the third person, and so on. The clay continues to be passed around the group until everyone accepts the finished product as a sign of God's love for us.

When no one wishes to make any more changes, call the large group back together and continue with these or similar words:

> When an individual's ideas come into contact with those of other people, the result is usually a shift, modification or change in those ideas. In this activity your ideas have been molded and remolded as the clay passed from hand to hand. What were you trying to express by the model your small group formed? How did you feel when others changed or modified your idea? How well does this final sign or symbol express what you wished to express?

Invite sharing on these questions.

My Ideas about the Sacraments

PURPOSE

To give participants an opportunity to reflect upon and share their thoughts about the sacraments.

MATERIALS NEEDED

- One pencil for each participant
- Activity Sheet K, one copy for each participant, copied on two separate sheets (see pp. 143–44)

DIRECTIONS

A word of caution is necessary with this activity. If the leader has reason to believe that a majority of the people in the group know virtually nothing about sacraments (for example, if they come from non-Christian or non-sacramental traditions), then this activity would not be appropriate.

The purpose of this exercise is not to "test" people or to teach which are the correct answers but to give the leaders and sponsors a sense of what people think about the sacraments and to help identify the areas that need to be emphasized or clarified.

Have each participant fill out Activity Sheet K. Read the directions aloud and make sure everyone understands what is to be done. Allow sufficient time for all to finish the entire exercise.

Then ask participants to form small groups and to share any answers they crossed off and why. Then for each sacrament take a count of the number of votes received by each "correct" answer. Discuss what is suggested by the fact that various people rated the answers differently.

While the discussion takes place, one of the leaders should collect the participants' questions about God and combine those that are similar. If there is time, answer those questions you can and answer the remaining questions later, either in the group or individually, as appropriate.

6.

ACTIVITIES ABOUT THE EUCHARIST

For Catholics, the entire Christian life focuses on the Eucharist. Therefore, it is imperative that participants understand and appreciate that the Lord becomes present among us in the simple staples of life, bread and wine. The following three activities can be used to introduce the church's teachings on the Eucharist and to help people to appreciate the fitness of bread and wine as our spiritual food and drink.

Taste and See

Purpose

To enable participants to *experience* the appropriateness of bread (and wine) as the material of the Eucharist.

Materials needed

- Enough hearty whole wheat bread for each participant to have a piece
- (Optional) Enough wine for each participant to have a very small portion

Directions

Give a piece of bread to each participant and invite everyone to examine the bread silently. Ask them to look intently at the bread and then to smell it and feel it. Finally, invite them to taste a piece, chewing it carefully and savoring it.

When all have finished, ask them to describe to the entire group what they saw, smelled, felt and tasted as they examined the bread. Then ask how they felt doing this exercise and what memories it brought to mind. Finally, ask them to share in what way this experience of bread reminds them of God's part in their life.

The process may be repeated with small glasses of wine.

Celebrating Community

PURPOSE

To bring to the participants' attention the elements of any good celebration.

MATERIALS NEEDED

- None

DIRECTIONS

Ask the participants to form small groups in which each person in turn talks about his or her favorite family celebrations: who attends, what food and drink is served and what rituals or activities or games are usually part of the celebration. When all have had a chance to share, reassemble everyone and discuss:

- how people feel when they attend such celebrations
- what happens to the relationships among the people who attend these celebrations.

The answers to these questions offer an opportunity to lead into an exposition of the characteristics of any good liturgy and an explanation of the idea behind the Eucharist.

What Is the Eucharist?

PURPOSE

To surface the basic *thoughts* and *ideas* participants have about the Eucharist.

MATERIALS NEEDED

- One pencil for each participant
- Activity Sheet L, one copy for each participant, copied on two separate sheets (see pp. 145–46)
- Chalkboard or newsprint
- Chalk or marker

DIRECTIONS

Introduce this exercise with these or similar words:

> There are many ways of thinking about the Eucharist. This exercise is designed to help us share our ideas with each other. Remember that the purpose of this activity is not to correct or contradict each other but to listen and learn together.

Have each participant fill out Activity Sheet L. Read the directions aloud and make sure everyone understands what is to be done. Allow sufficient time for all to finish the entire exercise.

Then in the large group go through each of the ten statements and ask the participants how they rated each statement. List the number who mostly or totally disagreed. Review each statement that had a large amount of disagreement and ask those who disagreed to explain why. Then ask the others to respond. Do not try to reach any firm conclusions.

While the discussion takes place, one of the leaders should collect the participants' questions about the Eucharist and combine those that are similar. If there is time, answer those questions you can and answer the remaining questions later, either in the group or individually, as appropriate.

7.

ACTIVITIES ABOUT PRAYER

Prayer is essential to the spiritual journey. People generally tend to equate prayer with petitions, but there are also prayers of praise, contrition and thanksgiving.

Those with some Catholic background may identify prayer with set formulas. Those without such a background may be more accustomed to spontaneous prayer. Some will have made some form of meditation or contemplative prayer a part of their regular prayer life. Finally, all will be familiar with some form of public worship as prayer.

These four activities may be used at any point during the initiation process. You might use all of them, each at a different stage. In any case, participants need to be assured that whatever praying they have done or are doing is good, but that there are also some other ways of praying which they may wish to try and might find helpful.

Ways to Pray

PURPOSE

To make participants conscious of the way they have prayed at different times of their lives.

MATERIALS NEEDED

- One pencil for each participant
- Activity Sheet M, one copy for each participant (see p. 147)

DIRECTIONS

Begin the activity with these or similar words:

> There are many different ways to pray. Some of us were taught to recite certain *formula* prayers, such as the Hail Mary or the Act of Contrition. Others may have discovered the beauty of *spontaneous* prayer, where we talk directly to God in our own words. Some may have even experienced the discipline of *meditation* or *contemplative* prayer, which attempts to go beyond words and lift the spirit into direct contact with God. Finally, public *worship,* such as the Mass and other liturgies are also a form of prayer. All of these methods are good, and each has its own strengths and weaknesses.
>
> The following exercise will help us identify the various ways we have prayed at different times in our lives.

Have each participant fill out Activity Sheet M. Read the directions aloud and make sure everyone understands what is to be done. Allow sufficient time for all to finish the entire exercise.

Then ask the participants to share their charts in small groups and to comment on them by discussing these questions:

> Do you see any pattern in your chart?
>
> Why do you think you prayed as you did at these times?
>
> What mix of methods of prayer would you like to achieve, and why?

A sample completed Activity Sheet might look like this:

	Childhood	Adolescence	Young Adult (18-30)	Adult (30-60)	Older Adult (60+)
Formula	50 %	90 %	10 %	5 %	%
Spontaneous	40 %	0 %	90 %	5 %	%
Meditation	5 %	0 %	0 %	40 %	%
Worship	5 %	10 %	0 %	50 %	%
Total	100%	100%	100%	100%	100%

Types of Prayer

PURPOSE

To give participants an opportunity to identify and experience different types of prayer.

MATERIALS NEEDED

- One pencil for each participant
- One sheet of paper for each participant
- Four pictures that evoke the four types of prayer

DIRECTIONS

Introduce this exercise with these or similar words:

> Most of us are familiar with prayer as *petition*. For example, we ask God in the Our Father to "give us this day our daily bread." But there are other types of prayer, such as *praise*, in which we glorify God, *contrition*, in which we ask God for forgiveness, and *thanksgiving*, in which we thank God for specific blessings.
>
> This simple activity will help us identify—and perhaps even experience—each of these four types of prayer.

First, hold up the four pictures one at a time and invite the participants to say a brief, silent prayer as they look at each one. When you have finished, ask them what type of prayer (praise, contrition, petition, thanksgiving) came to their minds as they looked at each picture, and why.

Then ask everyone to use one of the pictures as a basis for composing any one of the four types of prayer. They should write their prayers down on the sheets of paper. When they are finished, invite those who wish to share the prayers they have composed with the entire group.

Conclude by pointing out that different pictures evoked different types of prayer from different people, based on where each person is in his or her life at the present time.

Praying to Whom?

Purpose

To make participants more conscious of how the object or recipient of their prayers changes.

Materials needed

- One pencil for each participant
- Activity Sheet N, one copy for each participant (see p. 149)

Directions

Have each participant fill out Activity Sheet N. Read the directions aloud and make sure everyone understands what is to be done. Allow sufficient time for all to finish the entire exercise.

Then ask participants to share their charts in the smaller groups and discuss why they think the recipient of their prayer changed at different times in their lives.

A completed Activity Sheet might look like this:

Childhood	Adolescence	Young Adult (18–30)	Adult (30–60)	Older Adult (60+)
Guardian Angel	Jesus	God the Father	God	
God		MARY	Holy Spirit	
St. Joseph				

My Experience of Prayer

Purpose

To surface the participants' *feelings* and *questions* about prayer.

Materials needed

- One pencil for each participant
- Activity Sheet O, one copy for each participant, copied on two separate sheets (see pp. 151–52)

Directions

Have each participant fill out Activity Sheet O. Read the directions aloud and make sure everyone understands what is to be done. Allow sufficient time for all to finish the entire exercise.

Then invite participants to form small groups to share and discuss the reasons for their answers. Assure them that in the sharing they need not reveal any answer that would embarrass them or make them feel uneasy.

When they have finished, call the entire group together and invite them to share what insights about prayer surfaced during the discussion.

While the discussion takes place, one of the leaders should collect the participants' questions about prayer and combine those that are similar. If there is time, answer those questions you can and answer the remaining questions later, either in the group or individually, as appropriate.

8.

ACTIVITIES ABOUT MORAL CHOICES

It is one thing to know what the church teaches about morality. It is another to accept these teachings, and still another to follow them. To prepare the group to hear the church's teachings, it is important to help them realize that making moral decisions involves a good deal of difficulty.

These two activities are designed to help participants identify the moral choices they face and raise any questions they might have about them.

A Rock and a Hard Place

PURPOSE

To dramatize the difficulty of making moral choices.

MATERIALS NEEDED

- One rough piece of rock for each participant

DIRECTIONS

Hand out the pieces of rock and introduce the activity by telling the entire group that different people look at rocks or stones from different perspectives. Then ask the group how the following people might look at their rock and what they might do with it:

a geologist

a jeweler or gemologist

a miner

an architect

a construction contractor

a little boy sitting by a pond.

Continue the activity with these or similar words:

> Michelangelo looked at a piece of uncut marble and said that he already saw the finished statue in it. All he had to do was take away the marble that hid the figure from view. Look at your piece of rock. Imagine it as large or as small as you wish. What figure do you see in it?

Allow each person time to share his or her reflection, then continue:

> The rock represents a hard moral decision you have to make or have had to make in the past. Find some characteristics of the rock which remind you of that decision—the color, the roughness or smoothness, the shape, the sharp angles, anything about the rock which suggests an aspect of your decision.

Then ask the people to form small groups and share:

what the decision is or was

how their particular rock is like the decision

what made the decision difficult

how they felt when facing the decision

how they feel at the present time about the decision they made or are about to make.

When the discussions are finished, have everyone put his or her rock in one pile in the middle of the room. Then form a circle around the pile, join hands and say the Lord's Prayer together.

Moral Choices

PURPOSE

To help participants identify their basic *ideas* regarding morality.

MATERIALS NEEDED

- One pencil for each participant
- Activity Sheet P, one copy for each participant, copied on two separate sheets (see pp. 153–54)

DIRECTIONS

Have each participant fill out Activity Sheet P. Read the directions aloud and make sure everyone understands what is to be done. Allow sufficient time for all to finish the entire exercise.

Then invite participants to form small groups and compare their answers. Ask each small group to formulate one question about the statement over which they disagreed the most.

Then ask each small group to present its question to the entire gathering so that all might discuss possible answers.

While the discussion takes place, one of the leaders should collect the participants' questions about morality and combine those that are similar. If there is time, answer those questions you can and answer the remaining questions later, either in the group or individually, as appropriate.

SECTION III

Activity Sheets for Reproduction and Distribution

These activity sheets are for use with some of the preceding activities. They are perforated for easy removal and may be reproduced for the participants. Where there are two sides, they should be copied on two separate sheets.

ACTIVITY SHEET A

Recounting the Call

Think of the following questions as addressed to you personally. Answer each question in the box provided.

1. In the book of Genesis we read that our first parents hid from God and that God came looking for them. "The Lord God called to the man and asked him, 'Where are you?' " (Gen. 3:9). How would you answer that question about where you are at present in your search for God?

2. Our search for God is God's work. It does not depend upon our own efforts, although we have to respond to the overtures that God makes to us. When the Jews murmured because Jesus told them that he was the bread of life, Jesus said, "No one can come to me unless the Father who sent me draws them" (John 6:44). What events in your life appear to be drawing you to God and/or to Jesus?

3. After Jesus had been identified by John the Baptist as the Lamb of God, two of his disciples began to walk after Jesus. Jesus turned to them and asked, "What are you looking for?" (John 1:38) Today you need to answer similar questions. What are you looking for from Jesus? What are you looking for from the Catholic Church? What are you looking for from this group of people?

4. What difference do you think it will make to your life if you find what you are looking for?

ACTIVITY SHEET B

My Ideas about Church

Circle the number closest to your idea of church.

1=Agree completely / 2=Agree mostly / 3=Do not know

4=Disagree mostly / 5=Disagree completely

Jesus wanted all people to belong to one church.	1 2 3 4 5
It makes little difference to which church you belong.	1 2 3 4 5
All churches teach pretty much the same thing.	1 2 3 4 5
Being Catholic is a matter of doing the right thing.	1 2 3 4 5
Being Catholic is a matter of believing the right truths.	1 2 3 4 5
Being Catholic is a way of life.	1 2 3 4 5
The church is the mystical Body of Christ.	1 2 3 4 5
The church is the Pope, bishops, priests and religious.	1 2 3 4 5
The church is the pilgrim people of God.	1 2 3 4 5
The church is me.	1 2 3 4 5

Questions about the Catholic Church that I have:

Name (optional) ______________________________

ACTIVITY SHEET C

We All Need One Another

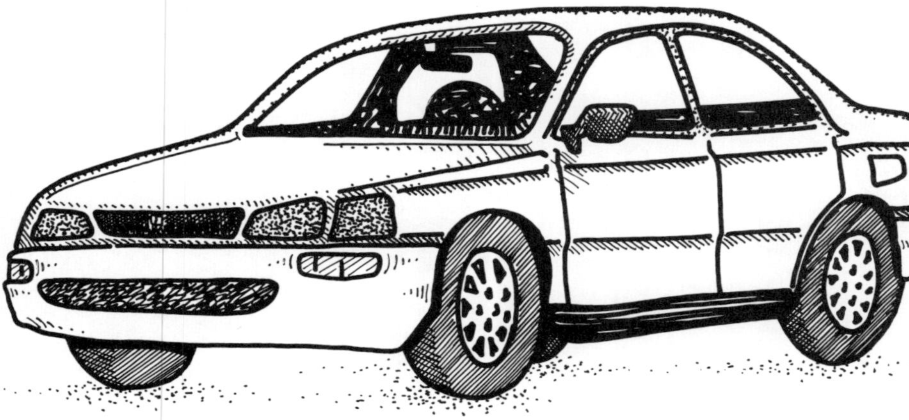

Among the parts of the car, I could choose to be the: engine, spark plugs, air filter, oil filter, gas, oil, chassis, frame, doors, windshield, seats, brakes, transmission, electrical system, battery, lights, wheel lugs, fan, fan belt, cooling system, tires, wheels, steering wheel, rear view mirror, carburetor, gas tank, bumper, springs, shock absorbers, horn, trunk, pistons, hubcap, directional indicator, radio, defogger.

I would like to be ______________________________

because ______________________________

____

Example:

I would like to be *a door*

because *I will protect my fellow journeyers from falling out and getting injured.*

ACTIVITY SHEET D

Old and New Wine Skins

Surround each wine skin with the ideas/behavior listed.

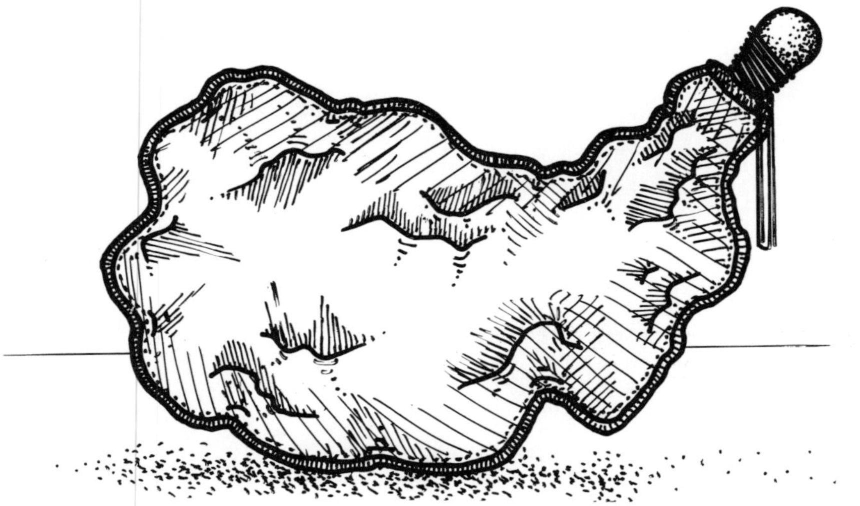

Old ideas/behavior I have had to put away.

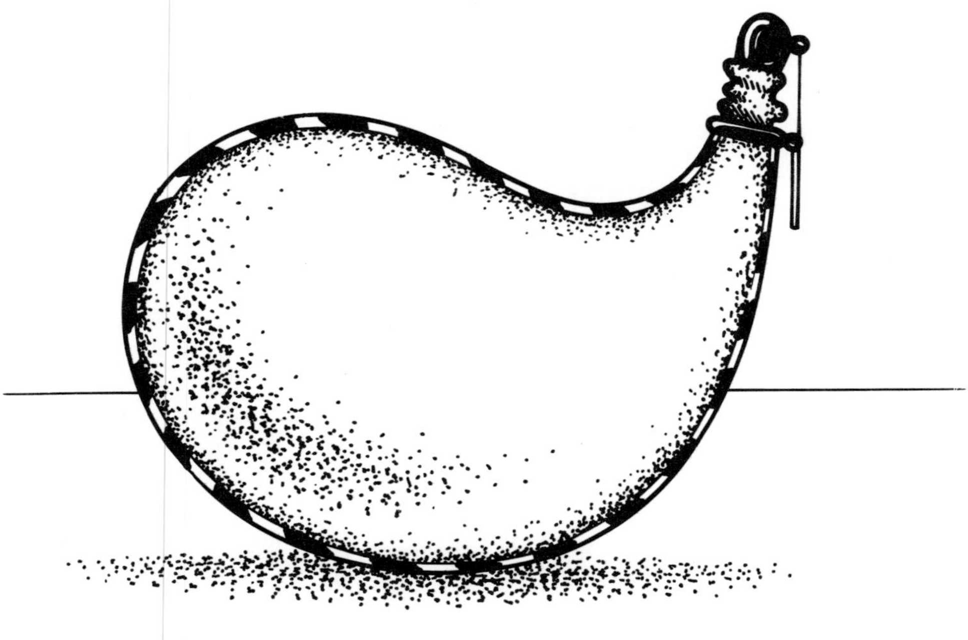

New ideas/behavior I have acquired.

ACTIVITY SHEET **E**

My Ideas about God

Circle the dot between each set of responses indicating the strength of your ideas about God. For example, if you completely agree with one statement, circle the dot right next to that statement; if you have no opinion at all, or think either statement could be true, circle the dot halfway between the two statements.

God:

is within all things • • • • • is in heaven.

never changes • • • • • changes frequently.

is interested in each thing I do • • • • • is interested only in some lthings I do.

has a definite plan for my life • • • • • has only a general plan for my life.

punishes people • • • • • allows people to suffer the effects of their own decisions.

is all-forgiving • • • • • is angry.

looks upon me as a sinner • • • • • looks upon me as a beloved child.

is indifferent to me • • • • • is vitally concerned about me.

can be pictured • • • • • cannot be pictured in any way.

is a father • • • • • is a mother.

Questions I have about God:

Name (optional)____________________________________

ACTIVITY SHEET F

The Roots of My Faith

On the tree on the other side, indicate:

On the **two large tap roots:** your mother's and your father's religions.

On the **next largest roots**: the predominant religions of your ancestors, as far back as you know them.

On the **smallest roots**: the religions of other people—friends, co-workers, relatives—who have had a significant impact on your religious beliefs and practices.

On the **limbs and leaves**: religious ideas and practices you have acquired from others; for example, concepts of God, Jesus, church, or habits of prayer or good works. Use the branches for things that were strong and persisted, and the leaves for those not so powerful.

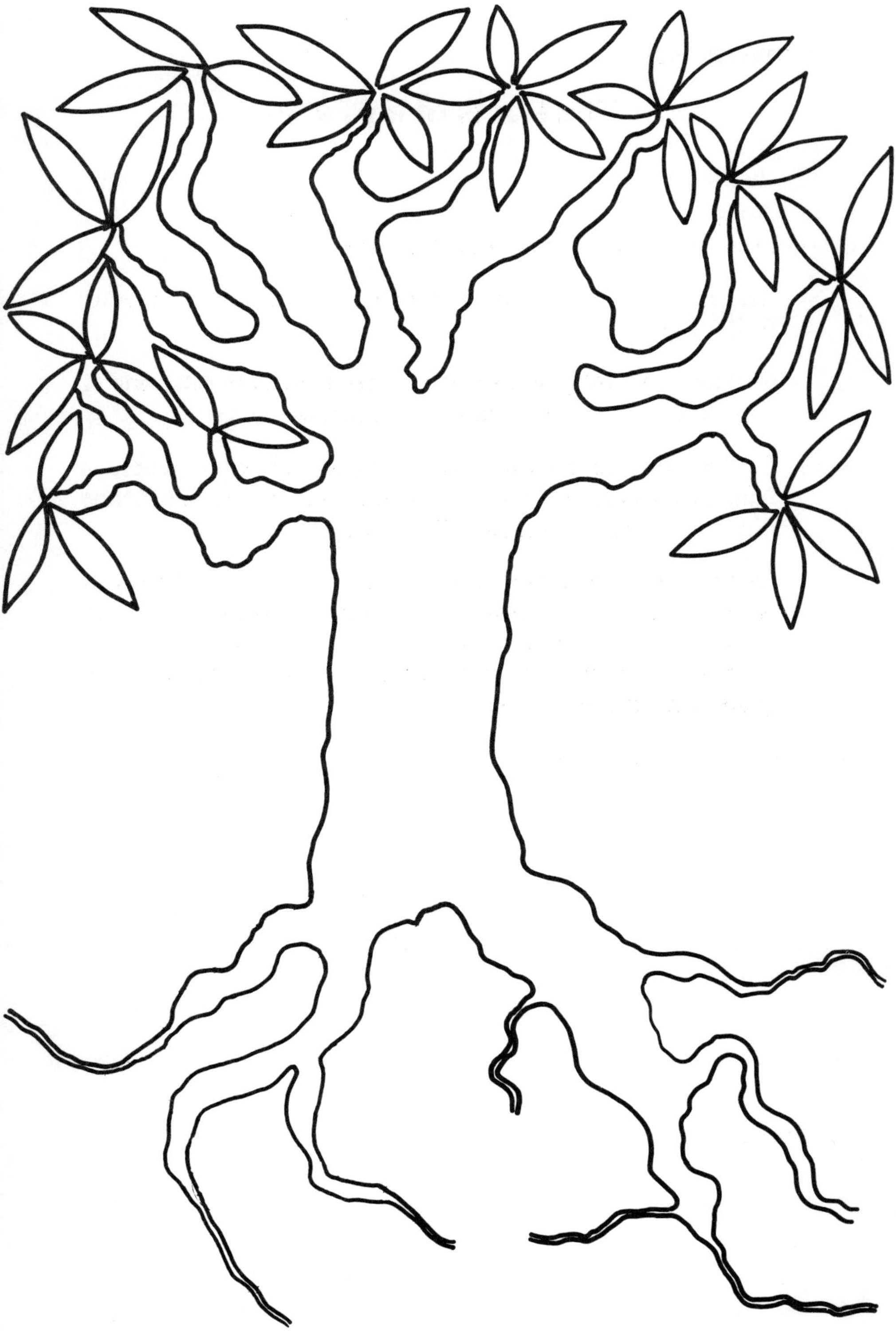

ACTIVITY SHEET G

What I Believe about the Bible

Circle the dot that is closest to what you believe. (The middle dot means you have no opinion.)

The Bible:

is the literal word of God	• • •	God's ideas in human words
was written over many centuries	• • •	was written at one time
is historically accurate in all details	• • •	is generally accurate
is a library of books	• • •	is one book
is not meant to be a science book	• • •	is scientifically accurate
contains all the same type of literature	• • •	contains many different types of literature
is a detailed guide on how to live	• • •	is a general guide on how to live
helps us understand God	• • •	helps us understand humans

The Old Testament:

is the story of the Jews	• • •	is prophecy about Jesus
is not that important in helping us today	• • •	is very important in helping us today

Questions I have about the Bible:

Name (optional) ________________________________

ACTIVITY SHEET H

How I Came to Know Jesus

Answer each question in the box provided:

How and when did you come to know Jesus?
When you were a child, who was the most influential person in forming your image of Jesus ?
Who or what has been the most influential person or event in forming your image of Jesus since you became an adult?

ACTIVITY SHEET I

Who Is Jesus Christ?

Mark each statement "T" for true, "F" for false, "?" for not sure.

Jesus was as human as we are.	______
Jesus sometimes broke the Jewish law.	______
Jesus right now is no longer human.	______
Jesus often preached against sexual sins.	______
Jesus is alive today.	______
Jesus knew all things when he was a child.	______
Jesus was not a revolutionary in any sense.	______
Jesus still has human consciousness and human feelings.	______
Jesus taught a morality different from the Ten Commandments.	______
Jesus saw the world from a male perspective.	______
Jesus liked some people better than others.	______
Jesus had feelings of anger, fear and affection.	______
Jesus taught religious doctrines.	______
Jesus looked and acted like a man, but he really was God inside.	______
Jesus grew as a person through the affection and guidance of his parents.	______
Jesus is the same today as he was when he walked in Palestine.	______
Seeing and knowing Jesus is seeing and knowing God the Father.	______
Jesus asked people to change their view of themselves and of life.	______
Jesus made a free decision to die on the cross.	______
The New Testament is an accurate historical biography of Jesus.	______

Questions I have about Jesus:

Name (optional)____________________________________

ACTIVITY SHEET J

The Church Is Like . . .

Circle only one word from each pair that best reflects your impressions of the church. Do not wrestle with the exact symbolism of each word. Go with your *feeling*. If you cannot choose, skip to the next pair of words.

The church is more like a		than a
1.	rose	daisy
2.	station wagon	motorcycle
3.	lump of clay	piece of steel
4.	tree	vine
5.	shoe	glove
6.	bat	ball
7.	hammer	saw
8.	eagle	hen
9.	knife	fork
10.	sheet of paper	pen
11.	body of water	mass of air
12.	pyramid	circle
13.	phone conversation	answering machine
14.	dog	lion
15.	radio station	bank

Questions I have about the church:

Name (optional ______________________________

ACTIVITY SHEET **K**

My Ideas about the Sacraments

Most of the following statements are correct, but for each sacrament circle only that *one* that is closest to what you think is the main purpose of the sacrament. In addition, if you think any of the statements is *false*, cross it out.

1. Baptism is . . .
   the way a person joins the church
   the moment in which a person receives the Holy Spirit
   necessary for salvation
2. Confirmation is . . .
   a reconfirming of Baptism
   a conferring of the Holy Spirit
   a part of initiation into the church
   a designation as a soldier of Christ
3. Eucharist is . . .
   a perfect way of giving thanks to God
   a way of remembering the dying and rising of Christ
   Jesus present under the forms of bread and wine
4. Reconciliation is . . .
   having our sins forgiven
   renewing our relationship with God
   repairing our relationship with the church
   necessary to have serious sins forgiven
5. Anointing of the Sick is . . .
   preparation for death
   a prayer for healing
   comfort for the sick
   forgiveness of sin
6. Matrimony is . . .
   the uniting of a couple with Christ
   a permanent lifelong commitment
   a call from God
   a way to live the Gospel
7. The task of those in Holy Orders is . . .
   primarily preaching
   primarily celebrating the Eucharist
   primarily guiding the parish
   primarily forgiving sins

Questions I have about the sacraments:

Name (optional) ______________________________

ACTIVITY SHEET L

What Is the Eucharist?

To the left of each statement write the number that best corresponds with your thoughts:

1=Agree completely / 2=Agree mostly / 3=Do not know

4=Disagree mostly / 5=Disagree completely

___1. The bread and wine literally *become* the body and blood of Jesus.

___2. The bread and wine are only symbols of Jesus.

___3. The Eucharist should be the most important thing in a Christian's life.

___4. Christians should receive communion every Sunday.

___5. After the Mass is finished, Jesus remains truly present in the bread and wine.

___6. The reading of the scriptures and the homily are the most important parts of the Mass.

___7. During the Mass is a good time for saying my personal, private prayers.

___8. We should not touch the Eucharist with our hands as a sign of respect.

___9. We need to receive both bread and wine to fully receive Jesus.

___10. Something else could be substituted for bread and wine in the Eucharist if it were done respectfully and in good taste.

Questions I have about the Eucharist are:

Name (optional) ______________________________________

ACTIVITY SHEET **M**

Ways to Pray

Reflect on the various ways you have prayed at different stages of your life. Assign a rough percentage of your prayer life to each method for each period. (Of course, only fill out the chart up to the present stage of your life.)

	Childhood	Adolescence	Young Adult (18–30)	Adult (30–60)	Older Adult (60+)
Formula	%	%	%	%	%
Spontaneous	%	%	%	%	%
Meditation	%	%	%	%	%
Worship	%	%	%	%	%
Total	100%	100%	100%	100%	100%

ACTIVITY SHEET N

Praying to Whom?

For each stage in your life, list the primary person or persons to whom your prayers were addressed. (Of course, only fill out the chart up to the present stage of your life.)

Childhood	Adolescence	Young Adult (18–30)	Adult (30–60)	Older Adult (60+)

Examples:

God

God the Father

Jesus

The Holy Spirit

Guardian Angel

A favorite saint

The Blessed Mother

Note: Non-Christians might have other names or images for the recipients of their prayers.

ACTIVITY SHEET O

My Experience of Prayer

Mark the following statements "A" (always), "O" (often), "S" (seldom), "N" (never), based on your own experience.

____ 1. My prayers are heard.

____ 2. Prayer is an important part of my daily routine.

____ 3. My prayers are set formulas.

____ 4. My prayers are spontaneous.

____ 5. I meditate or use contemplative prayer.

____ 6. I pray through church services or public worship.

____ 7. I pray about the daily events of my life.

____ 8. I feel close to God whenever I pray.

____ 9. I have a great many distractions when I pray.

____ 10. I receive answers to my prayers.

Questions I have about prayer are:

Name (optional)____

ACTIVITY SHEET **P**

Moral Choices

Mark the following statements "A" (agree), "D" (disagree), "U" (unsure).

____ 1. Morality is a relationship with God, rather than a set of rules.

____ 2. What I think is right or wrong makes an action moral or not.

____ 3. Growth in moral maturity only comes from taking risks and asking questions.

____ 4. The church should not speak out on questions of business practices or government policies.

____ 5. In making moral decisions, one should look for guidance exclusively from the Bible.

____ 6. In making moral decisions, one should look for guidance exclusively from the church.

____ 7. A decision which I think is morally good may be a serious mistake or even harmful to myself or others.

____ 8. The Christian moral code is very restrictive.

____ 9. The Christian moral code is very liberating.

____ 10. The church makes too many rules.

____ 11. The church does not make enough rules.

____ 12. Morality is concerned primarily with what is sinful or not sinful.

Questions I have about morality are:

Name (optional) ____________________________________